MEDICINE AND YOU: IS IT A GOOD FIT? A DOCTOR'S PERSPECTIVE

Dr Mudit Kumar,
MD, FRCPCH

CONTENTS

INTRODUCTION

This book is intended for primarily high school, higher
secondary, A level or IB students who are interested in pursuing a career in the medical field. These students are starting to make important decisions about their future career paths and may be actively exploring different career options.

The book can also be valuable for other individuals involved in supporting high school students in their career exploration journey.

This can include parents, teachers, guidance counselors, and mentors who play a role in guiding and advising students on their career choices. These individuals can also benefit from gaining insights into the medical field and understanding how to best support students who are considering a career in medicine.

As I have also covered in this book, various specialities of medicine, what its like working in those, after completing the training whether you should work for yourself or some one else, taking career break, research and finally retirement, this book will also act as valuable source of inside information for current medical graduates.

PREFACE

UNVEILING THE INK: THE PASSION, PURPOSE, AND JOURNEY BEHIND WRITING THIS BOOK

Reasons I choose to write this book are many but some of the important ones are to share my experiences from being a high school student to becoming a doctor and being in this profession for nearly four decades. I have seen medicine changing phenomenally over these many years and particularly in the last few years and now with the advent of Artificial Intelligence and Machine learning I think it's going to change dramatically in the next few years.

I entered medical school nearly forty years ago and am currently practicing as a consultant, pediatrician and neonatologist. Now you must be wondering why it took so long for me to write this book. I hope after reading this book you will understand why right from entering medical school to practicing medicine as a career a doctor hardly finds any time to pursue any other interest outside medicine.

This is my attempt to help the students who are still debating, whether to choose medicine as a career or not. This is a million dollar question in the students mind and I will try to make it easier for them to answer this question.

As a High School student, on lots of occasions, you must be thinking what is the best way to unleash your potential, unlock your future and create your own destiny. Sometimes we have very unrealistic ambitions or goals in our life but believe it or not these do help in becoming very successful in your future career

I'll give my example when I was in High School and even as a kid I was crazy about the movies but I did not want to become an actor rather I wanted to direct the movies, wanted to learn the tricks and art of directing a movie through proper channel or going to a proper Institute rather than doing straight apprenticeship and jumping into cinema. I spent my childhood in India where people are crazy about movies more than any other country and there used to be a very famous college called Film and Television Institute in Pune. When I was in class 12th which is the time when you chose to apply either for medicine or engineering which used to be the two major professions or in fact only two to choose from if you want to get a secured job and career. You can only choose one or the other and most parents would like their children in India to take either of these options and in fact students and parents could not even think of a third option.

But as I mentioned that I wanted to become a film director so I contacted this Film and Television Institute and at that time everything was done via the post and they sent me an application form to apply for the course which I think was for two years and you can go straight into that after finishing your High School. I filled that application form but it needed a signature from the parents so I had to tell my parents and that was the first time I told my parents that I want to go into the films. My father was a doctor himself so his expectation was that I should only and only choose to become a doctor and as a student I was quite good in studies, he was pretty sure that I would compete and pass the entrance exam to go into medicine. So this news came as a shock to him and he became very upset that I am not thinking of choosing medicine as a career.

In those times we did not have counselors to help us and put us in the right direction and whether what we are thinking is the right decision. You can imagine and very well understand as you all may be of the same age group, that when you are 16-17 how mature your brain can be.

So I kept thinking and debating myself without discussing with anyone else. I was also not very open with my parents so I did not indulge in any kind of open discussion with them and finally decided that I will give up my dreams and go into medicine. I am still as crazy as I was about the movies and I haven't given up my dream to direct a movie or a small series on Netflix or similar platform during and even after retiring from medicine.

"You must follow your passion. You must follow your dreams. If you don't, you're throwing away the opportunity for greatness." - Scent of a Woman

It was funny that the reason I then decided to become a doctor was that I may be able to earn money quickly as a doctor by opening my own hospital and by that I can have enough money to make my own movie. Now thinking back sounds very silly and funny however that kind of unrealistic thinking helped me to decide that it's okay to go to medicine not only because my Dad wants to but because that will help get enough money to finance my own movie.

But the penny dropped when I entered medical school and very soon I realized that it's not as easy as I thought it was going to be and it's real hard work. Even when I passed out I realized that to establish yourself and to start earning the money it may take years of hard work and then eventually all my dreams of making movies vanished in thin air. Very soon I realized that the real word is very different from what

I thought

CHAPTER 1

THE SECRETS UNVEILED: A RIVETING GUIDE TO UNLOCKING YOUR CAREER IN MEDICINE

"Medicine is not just a profession; it's a calling to make a difference in the lives of others."

First of all I want to clarify that I am not a high school counselor and I'm not going to advise you which Medical School to choose and how to apply and do the application. Once you have decided that you want to go in medicine you will have lots of help and advice from professionals, your family members and most importantly your parents

What I am going to tell you in this book is as an insider in this profession, what my experience has been and how I have seen this profession changing so rapidly in terms of demand of the patients and also the technology and the treatment options. And how the newly qualified doctor has to keep pace with all these.

And I would also like to tell ups and downs of medical profession and I'll try not to be biased here but of course give my personal opinion and whether or not if given the choice and I can be high school student again would I choose to go to the medical school or not.

I have the privilege of practicing medicine and working as a doctor in three different countries, one developing Nation and two developed Nations so I feel that I am in a good position to compare the health care system and working in different countries with different health Economics.

The advice or discussions I will have here in this book will be relevant to the high school students across the world.

The world is changing fast and so is the medicine

If there is one profession in the world which I can think of which will never go out of fashion and will rather be a necessity, that undoubtedly is medicine.

With the emergence of new technology such as artificial Intelligence, the way the future generation will learn is going to be very different from what it used to be in our generation or in the current generation. However, I still feel that the profession of medicine will continue to follow fundamental core philosophy, that humans cannot be replaced by machines.

Although lots of people are skeptical about use of these technologies in medicine at the moment but there is strong argument that these will be beneficial and help doctors in looking after their patients in more efficient way and will also help in developing new ways of rapid diagnostic tests, newer forms of treatments and even new vaccines to fight against the infections.

CHAPTER 2

THE HEALING SYMPHONY: UNVEILING THE WONDERS OF THE MEDICAL PROFESSION AND ITS MULTIFACETED FIELDS

"The practice of medicine combines science, art, and the human connection, making it a truly fulfilling career."

Medical profession is one of the oldest professions in the world, dating back nearly 5000 years. The earliest description of medical treatment we have are from India China and Egypt

Who`s a doctor?

To me, doctor is like a superhero in a white coat, armed with a stethoscope instead of a cape. They have the magical ability to make you say "Ahh!" and ask you strange questions about your bodily functions.

Doctors are masters of deciphering the mysterious language of medical jargon and prescribing potions that may taste like a concoction from a witch's cauldron.

They can wield needles like tiny swords and perform tricks that would make a magician envious.

But let's not forget about the paperwork. Being a doctor is also like being a professional form-filler-outer. You have to document every symptom, every test, every diagnosis, every treatment. It's like playing a never-ending game of Scrabble.

But at the end of the day, being a doctor is also incredibly rewarding. You have the opportunity to make a real difference in people's lives, to heal their bodies and ease their pain. And that's no laughing matter.

When you go to medical school after finishing a graduate degree, which is the basic medical degree before choosing which kind of doctor you want to become and which field of medicine you want to specialize, it may very much depend on what kind of personality you have although the basic traits of being a good doctor remains the same. Still to become a successful and safe doctor in your chosen specialty It will help if your personality matches with the demand of that specialty.

To 'do no harm' is the ethical foundation of professionalism in medicine, which every doctor should follow, no matter which specialty of medicine they decide to choose.

As an important step in becoming a doctor, medical students must take the Hippocratic Oath. And one of the promises within that oath is "first, do no harm" (or "primum non nocere," the Latin translation from the original Greek.)

This is part of the Hippocratic oath which the doctors still take during their graduation ceremony in most of the countries although in a lot of countries for example in the USA a modified version is used. Recently lots of doctors have raised ethical questions whether or not they should take the oath as now in all the countries their professional conduct is monitored by regulating authorities.

I have to say that it's quite fun taking the oath along with all your batch mates in front of your family and parents and it also gives you a sense of accomplishment and you feel like society has given you a responsibility. Remember people in public are looking at you as a responsible member of the society whose code of conduct is higher than any other profession because you're also taking an oath.

Attributed to the Greek physician and teacher Hippocrates of Kos, who is often called the Father of medicine, the true author of the oath is unknown, and in fact there may have been several authors.

After Greek political power fell and the influence of the Hippocratic school faded, the oath fell into obscurity for nearly 2000 years. It was rediscovered by medieval Christian scholars and in 1508 was used in a ceremony at the University of Wittenberg. By 1750 the Hippocratic oath had been translated into English and other European languages, and for several centuries a version of the oath was recited by graduating doctors.

As the practice of medicine has changed so have the oaths taken. One of the most significant revisions was first drafted in 1948 by the World Medical Association (WMA), called the Declaration of Geneva.

"Remember, every journey starts with a single

*step. Pursuing a career in medicine is your first
step towards a world of endless possibilities."*

Which branch of medicine you should choose to specialize in, first of all should be based on your interest and what kind of specialist you want to become. Considering the fact that this is what you are going to do in your professional career for the rest of your life. So choose the specialty you will enjoy and be comfortable and happy in practicing.

Most people will divide their interest broadly into two categories: either you want to go into surgical specialties or you do not want to go into surgical specialties. Depending on how you feel your hand skill coordination are and whether you are happy to use scalpel and scissors on your patients to relieve them of their pain and suffering. If you do not like being inside the operating theater or would rather prefer to make a challenging diagnosis and treat your patients with medications then opt for non-surgical specialty.

In medicine we provide three Levels of care to our patients. These are called Primary, Secondary and Tertiary care. Primary care is mainly provided by the family physicians or general physicians the name varies from one country to another for example in the US they are known as Family Physicians whereas in the UK they are known as GPs or General Physicians.

Secondary care doctors practice different specialties

of medicine for example to name a few they are called Surgeons, Physicians, Pediatricians, Orthopedicians, Obstetricians.

The tertiary level of care is provided by the doctors who super specialize for example, Pediatric Gastroenterologist who deal with children only with gut problems or a Heart surgeons who deals with the patients who come with the heart attack and needs operation or children who are born with heart defects and need operation without which they may even die.

The pathway generally followed is that a primary care physician will refer the patients to the secondary care physicians and secondary care physicians to the tertiary level of physicians if needed.

From out-patients or clinics doctors will refer the patients for admission to the hospital under the care of hospital physicians for admission called in-patient stay. These are the patients who cannot be managed in out-patients settings for example if they are too sick, they need continuous and close monitoring of their heart rate, oxygen levels, need intravenous fluids, intravenous antibiotics, certain tests which can only be done as in-patient and so on

> *"It is not our abilities that show what we truly are. It is our choice." - Harry Potter and the Chamber of Secrets*

I will touch on some of the mainstream and major specialties, one by one.

Surgery is a specialty which involves the use of manual or instrumental techniques to diagnose, treat, and manage various diseases, injuries, or conditions. It often involves invasive procedures where incisions are made to access and operate on the affected area of the body.

Every specialty of medicine requires a different set of skills but surgeons in particular need a very different kind of skill set which includes a bright, eager mind, manual dexterity and physical skills for performing an operation as per the Royal College of surgeons of England.

Surgeons often work as part of a multidisciplinary team, collaborating with anesthesiologists, nurses, surgical assistants, and other healthcare professionals. To become a successful surgeon, you must not only be good with your eye-hand coordination but should also have excellent communication skills and be a team leader.

You may have heard that nowadays robots are used to perform surgeries which is only partly true as the fact is that robots themselves do not operate on the patients on their own as shown in some sci-fi movies but in fact in robotic surgeries, which are mostly the ones which require quite precision and in which human hands cannot perform a procedure as precisely as the robots, then the surgeon controls and guides the robot to do the procedure by using a handheld device which Is more or less similar to how you control a character or a weapon or a car in a video game by using hand held game controller.

Internal medicine, also known as general medicine or internal medicine, is a medical specialty that focuses on the prevention, diagnosis, and non-surgical treatment of adult diseases.

Internal medicine physicians, also called internists, have a broad knowledge base and expertise in managing a wide range of diseases and conditions that affect adults. They are often the first point of contact for adult patients seeking medical care.

Although now this specialty is replaced by Family medicine, also known as general practice or family practice. This is a medical specialty that provides comprehensive and continuous healthcare for individuals and families of all ages.

Internists are mostly based in the hospitals looking after the in-patients. They only look after the adults whereas Family medicine physicians manage patients of all ages but mainly in out-patient settings.

Family physicians build long-term relationships with their patients and provide continuity of care across the lifespan. They kind of become part of the patient's family as they see most members of the family, hence the term Family medicine physicians.

They not only look after diseases and illness but also help their patients emotional, social, and psychological well-being. Family medicine physicians in a way become that family's mentor and guide as far as health is concerned.

Family medicine is one of the branches of medicine which has been there for thousands of years and is still very popular and in fact becoming increasingly popular. Family medicine physicians are in great demand across the world for the very reason that these doctors can help and manage a variety of medical conditions and they are the pillars of Primary Care.

Obstetrics and Gynecology, is a medical specialty that focuses on the care of pregnant women, childbirth, and the postpartum period. They also provide gynecological care, including routine exams, screenings, and treatments for conditions related to the female reproductive system.

Within Obstetrics, Fetal Medicine is becoming increasingly popular amongst new Obstetric trainees as it does not involve generally out of hours on-calls. Fetal medicine is a super specialization, done after finishing the core obstetrics and gynecology training. Fetal medicine involves diagnosing and managing fetal abnormalities and performing procedures such as prenatal diagnostic testing, fetal ultrasound, and fetal interventions, for example doing a surgical procedure even before the baby is born for life threatening conditions. This requires years of training and expertise.

Pediatrics and Neonatology are medical specialties that focus on the care of infants, children, and adolescents. Neonatologists specialize in the care of newborn infants, particularly those who are premature, have low birth weight, or have medical complications. They provide specialized medical and developmental care in neonatal intensive care units (NICUs) to promote optimal outcomes for newborns.

This is the specialty in which I am trained, it's very close to my heart and I have really enjoyed managing tiny premature babies and children over the years. I can keep on talking about this specialty and can write a whole chapter on this.

Pediatrics is often compared with Veterinary medicine, as neither animals nor small kids can tell you what their symptoms are or even where the pain is and what's bothering them. They may even be scared to be examined. Managing an ill child is a completely different ball game as compared to managing an ill adult. It requires adaptability, examining the child as best as you can and taking every opportunity to do so by distracting them or playing with them.

As they cannot tell you exactly what's wrong with them,
Pediatricians need to be observant and meticulous in

their assessments and interpretations. And of course the art of history taken from the parents is also very important, but sometimes parents may not give you relevant history so you may have to ask leading questions.

So if you think you have all those skills and you are good at dealing with kids, you will enjoy this specialty. Pediatricians are the happiest doctors, various studies have shown that the incidence of depression is lowest amongst the Pediatricians as compared to the doctors in other specialties.

Orthopedic surgeons also called bone doctors by people, diagnose and treat musculoskeletal conditions and injuries. So like Surgeons, having excellent hand-eye coordination and manual dexterity is essential for performing intricate tasks during surgical interventions.

Orthopedic surgeons may perform long surgeries and spend extended periods on their feet during patient consultations and hospital rounds. Physical stamina is important to sustain the demanding nature of the profession and provide optimal patient care, and this is a very important fact to remember when choosing this specialty.

Ophthalmologists or the eye doctors diagnose and treat a wide range of eye conditions and diseases. They deal with the delicate and intricate structures of the eye, so more than in any surgical branch, it requires precise movements and excellent hand-eye coordination. Most of the time they use a microscope to do the surgery as the parts of the eyes they are operating on cannot be seen by naked eyes.

Ophthalmology is a rapidly evolving field with advancements in technology and surgical techniques. Being adaptable to new innovations and advancements is crucial for providing optimal patient care if you are planning to choose this specialty. These are doctors who give blind people vision to see the world by doing various surgical procedures, the most common one you may have heard called corneal transplant.

ENT surgeons deal with intricate structures and diseases of the ear, nose, and throat. This is also an ever growing specialty as far as helping the patients with hearing difficulties is concerned. Modern technological advances and surgical procedures are transforming the lives of the people with hearing deficits. You may have heard about something called Cochlear implants, which are electronic devices designed to provide a sense of sound to individuals with severe to profound hearing loss. Some ENT surgeons specialize and get trained in doing this procedure.

Doctors working in surgical specialties such as General surgery, Brain surgery, Heart surgery, Orthopedicians, ENT to name few are the ones which operate on the patients for various surgical problems and these doctors spend lots of time in operating theaters with full scrubs, masks and lots of gadgets with the lights focused on the site of operation of the patient.

One interesting fact I would like to share here about these lights used in Operating rooms is that it doesn't produces shadow, so even if a surgeon or the assistant`s hands comes on the way while operating on their patients, the stream of the light is not blocked because the way these lights are designed with the help of advancing technology which is helping doctors every day in improving the patient care.

Anesthesiology is a branch of medicine in which doctors help the patients and the surgeons to make any surgical procedure pain free by using different combinations of medications. Lots of these doctors also diversify and become intensivist which means they work in Intensive Care units and look after very sick patients where lots of them are on breathing machines called ventilators.

Radiologists are medical doctors who specialize in diagnosing and treating diseases and injuries using medical imaging techniques. They play a crucial role in the healthcare system by interpreting various imaging modalities, such as X-rays, CT scans, MRI scans, ultrasound, and nuclear medicine scans

The preferences of specialties chosen by doctors have changed a lot since my days. For example, Radiology was not in high demand and it was understandable as

Radiologists had limited gadgets to help clinicians to establish a diagnosis.

But over the years there has been dramatic technological advances and new machines and soft wares are being developed everyday by medical or biomedical engineering companies. For example only few years ago the neuro imaging machines such as MRI (Magnetic Resonance Imaging) could only pick up brain tumor which is more than three or five millimeters but now they can diagnose brain tumor as small as less than one millimeter which is a very good news for the patients and if you pick up the brain tumors when they are very small it's easier for the surgeon to remove it or they can be taken care by radiation or medications.

As the new technology and software comes, the previous ones become obsolete and it's exactly the same as your current mobile phone may become outdated in the next one or two years because the new phones will have a better camera, better processing and better storage which will tempt you to buy a newer version of your phone. Similarly the hospitals across the world have to keep investing and keep pace with the newer technology which of course increases the cost of healthcare which is a major issue in most of the countries.

Radiology is also one of the specialties in which technological advances are being put into practice on a daily basis. Use of artificial intelligence or machine learning in the near future is going to be a game changer in this specialty as it will help doctors to read and analyze the images of the patients more accurately and more precisely.

In spite of all the buzz and phobia around machines taking the jobs of radiologists, I don't think it will replace the radiologist as ultimately the reporting of these images has to be done by a doctor and not by a machine for medico-legal reasons.

Artificial Intelligence tools will analyze the data from thousands of patients with similar images and then lead to an algorithm which will suggest the most likely diagnosis. These tools will definitely act as a very efficient assistant to a radiologist to help and guide them to report these images in lesser periods of time with more accuracy, which eventually will help the clinicians in making the diagnosis in a short period of time.

Now going back to the Radiology as being one of the top and highly sought after specialty nowadays by the medical graduates you can understand that most of you are very tech oriented and like playing and exploring different gadgets, as compared to our times when there were very few gadgets and in that too in a very primitive stage.

The other reason why Radiology as a specialty is very popular is that it allows you to have a better work-life balance, as there are no emergencies to handle and there is no direct dealing with the patient although in the big hospital settings radiologist are on call which means they may be asked in the middle of the night by an emergency doctor to see the radiological images and give them there expert opinion but the difference from other specialties is that they can do this by sitting in front of high resolution computer screen at the comfort of their home and in fact lots of hospitals nowadays take the help of the radiologist who maybe even stationed in a different country.

In fact Radiology is one of the very few specialties where you can work remotely nowadays like in lots of other professions.

Radiologists are the doctors who do not see any patients at all but crucially they help the clinicians in establishing the diagnosis and further management.

Within this specialty there is a subspecialty called Interventional Radiology in which these highly trained doctors do very specialized procedures with extreme precision and this could be a specialty of choice for any of you who are ambidextrous and have very good fine motor skills.

In Interventional radiology, doctors not only interpret patients' medical images, but they also perform minimally invasive surgical procedures through small incisions in the body.

Radiology may not be your choice of your specialty however if you want to get involved with the patients directly and want to talk to them, take their medical history, examine them and want to take the challenges of making a diagnosis and then seeing the outcome of your intervention directly.

Another specialty which is gaining lots of popularity among medical graduates is Dermatology which is a specialty related to the skin conditions. The main reason it's getting more popular is because cosmetology is now an important component of this dermatology and of course people want to look beautiful and anti-aging treatment is now a billion dollar business.

More and more people around the world are looking for more anti-aging and beauty treatments and dermatologists are qualified healthcare professionals, who are offering therapies and treatments which are based on evidence and are scientifically proven. Dermatologists like any other doctor in other specialties have to adhere to strict regulations for these kinds of treatments which makes them more popular amongst the public as they trust doctors more than beauty therapists for the right reasons.

As Dermatology nowadays is highly sought after specialty you have to rank really high to get into the training program in Dermatology and Cosmetology, the other reason why you have to rank high to get into Dermatology is that, as compared to the other specialties like medicines surgery and pediatrics the number of training posts in Dermatology are limited.

Like Radiology in Dermatology you can have better

professional versus lifestyle balance as there are no dermatological emergencies, so you do not do any night on calls and basically you work only during the day time with your own convenience in out-patient settings.

Financially also both Radiology and Dermatology are quite rewarding.

Intensive Care units are full of medical gadgets. I have noticed that medical students get quite fascinated with these gadgets when they do electives in these intensive care units whether it's adult, children's or neonatal. They get intrigued and sometimes even overwhelmed to see so much medical equipment being used in one single patient to save their lives particularly when lots of these equipment use modern computer soft wares. Patients' heart rate, breathing rate, blood pressure and their oxygen saturation level can all be monitored continuously by using computer algorithms and soft wares. Intensive Care doctors are experts in operating these machines with the help of Biomedical engineers.

So as a medical student if you are quite into gadgets and technology, you may decide to become intensivist, that will be fantastic news as ICUs across the word need more intensivist and this demand has particularly increased during pandemic.

When medical students graduates start their training, before choosing to become Intensivist they do a Intensive Care rotation for about six months to get the experience and feel that how it is really in working in Intensive Care and some of them then decide not to become intensivist as they understand that working with medical equipment's and gadget is only a small part of managing critically ill patients and to become a good intensivist you need to have the kind of temperament, where you can handle the mental and physical stress easily and do not get upset with the outcome of the patients which is not always positive.

You should also be able to switch off yourself from your patients and the hospital once your shift is over and you go home. Otherwise you may not be able to enjoy your time with your family at home. So if you have this kind of personality or temperament by all means do become intensivist as the world needs doctors like you.

Psychiatry is also one of those specialties where you need a similar kind of temperament to be able to switch off yourself once you have finished seeing the patient and gone home. As psychiatrists see people with mental health problems every day, lots of these patients are mentally depressed and they come to you asking for help. It's not easy not to get involved emotionally with whatever is going on in their lives.

It's like we as an audience getting too involved emotionally with a particular character while watching a movie or the method actors who get into the skin of the character they are playing so deeply that it takes months after finishing the shooting of that movie to get out of that character which can affect the well-being of actors. Australian actor Heath Ledger who played the iconic character of Joker in movie The Dark Knight being a classic example.

Medicine is increasingly becoming more and more highly specialized. For example some of the Orthopedic surgeons will only manage the injury or the problem with the knee joint or the hand or the shoulder. It's good and makes perfect sense if these doctors are practicing in top tier cities of the world because they will mostly be taking the referral from their other Orthopedic colleagues for their expertise in one joint only. However if you working in smaller cities you must be able to see all kind of bone problems It also depends on your interest some doctors would preferred to be super specialized but some would prefer to see all kinds of patients

But remember that higher you go up in the pyramid you may not be able to see many patients but you will become better and better as you are only managing one part of the body which is also good for the patients who can benefit from your expertise and super specialization

I can give examples of my specialty which is Pediatrics and Neonatology, which is a specialization of medicine to become a children's and newborn`s doctor. Now we have some super specialists in that as well for example Pediatric Gastroenterologist who will only see the children with problem with the stomach, intestine or nutrition but even in that sub specialty now there are doctors who are getting trained and specializing in just one organ for example in liver and they are called pediatric Hepatologist.

Neonatologists like me only take care of very tiny premature babies who are admitted to Neonatal Intensive Care (NICU) which is the ICU designated only for high risk babies and babies who are born prematurely and could be just 500 gms at birth as compared to average birth weight of 3000 gms.

"Don't let anyone ever make you feel like you don't deserve what you want. Go for it." - 10 Things I Hate About You

So depending on your interest, as medicine is expanding rapidly and is becoming super super specialized, it gives you the choice to go on the top of the pyramid if you want to but that doesn't mean the doctors who are not super specializing are less competent or doing lesser job and in fact the doctors who can see all kind of patient ailments may have more opportunity to work in any part of the world, whether its rural area or a big city and they may attract more patients because they will see all kind of illnesses within their specialty

As far as job security Is concerned doctors have always been in demand and will remain in demand in many years to come. World will always need good quality doctors.

But how secure your job is will also vary from country to country. For example, one of the countries where I was trained, which is the UK, the health care system there is called National Health Services or NHS. In UK the number of students admitted to the medical school are always in proportion to the training programs available in NHS hospitals which means after graduating you have almost 100% chance to get into the training posts although some specialties might be oversubscribed and you may have to wait to get train in that particular sub specialty.

When you finish your training and become full-fledged sub specialist doctor you will have almost 100% chance of getting consultant post in one of the NHS hospitals because the training posts increase or decrease depending on the consultant jobs available over next year so there is a career and job planning in UK and in fact UK is producing less doctors from their medical school then the actually required to run the NHS and you must be reading a lot in the media about the problem currently NHS is facing because of the shortage of the doctors and in fact NHS has always been dependent on doctors from abroad for many years to run their health services.

But before doctor who have graduated from other countries and who want to work in UK have to pass an exam called PLAB which is highly competitive, before the licensing authority called General Medical Council

(GMC) can give a license to practice in UK

Similarly other European countries for example Germany is also now trying to hire doctors from other countries because they don't have enough own medical graduates to run their health care system

The US produces a substantial number of medical graduates, however there is a lot of disparity in the doctor population ratio from one part of the country to another and there is a shortage of doctors in remote rural areas of the country where they are relying on the foreign doctors. But like in UK or European countries, to enter into the US Healthcare system and to get the license to practice in US the doctors who are trained and have graduated outside US have to sit in an exam which is both theoretical and clinical and very competitive

CHAPTER 3

THE UNPRECEDENTED INTERLUDE: HOW COVID-19 ORCHESTRATED A GLOBAL RHAPSODY, FOREVER RESHAPING THE MEDICAL PROFESSION

"In every crisis, there is an opportunity." - Money Heist

S tep into the extraordinary era that unfolded before our eyes, as the world was gripped by the COVID-19 pandemic, forever altering the course of history and leaving an indelible mark on the medical profession.

Covid-19 pandemic is the biggest pandemic in the history of mankind. Until May 2023 according to the World Health Organization website nearly 800 million people had Covid-19 confirmed by the tests and nearly 7 million have died sadly but unfortunately this is not the end of COVID -19 pandemic. It doesn't look like it is going to go away soon so the numbers may keep on rising.

It's a strange coincidence that almost 100 years ago in year 1918 we had the biggest pandemic of that century called Spanish flu which affected nearly 500 million people which was almost one third of the world population at that time and killed between 50 to 100 million people. As we did not had the modern laboratory testing methods and there was no accurate data, this is just an estimate and is quite likely that these numbers may have been much higher. It was also due to a virus called influenza virus, from a particular strain named H1N1. COVID - 19 is also name given to a particular strain of virus from the family of viruses called Coronavirus

During COVID-19 Pandemic the world came to halt which never happened before in the history of mankind. This Pandemic did not spare any race or any country. Every country imposed strict lockdowns.

As human beings our brain is not programmed like most other mammals to just eat, sleep and reproduce. So our brain and body went into a kind of shock mode. It was not prepared at all to do nothing. But the human beings are very adaptable and that's why we are advanced and on the highest level of Animal kingdom

> *"We can't change the past, but we can always learn from it." - The Pursuit of Happyness*

Now the reason I brought all that up in the context of this discussion is whether or not you should choose medicine as a career, because COVID-19 pandemic has changed the world in many ways, particularly about our way of working. Lots of daily routines like shopping, meeting people either for work or personal reasons started to happen virtually over mobile phones or computers.

COVID-19 pandemic drastically changed the way

people in most professions will work and even though now there are no lockdowns most people still want to work remotely as they have seen the benefits of that all though lots of employers do not agree with that.

But there are certain professions which include emergency services such as firefighters, police, ambulance crew and of course doctors and nurses who cannot work remotely so you have to bear that in mind that no matter what happens in the world and what people in other professions are doing you have to be at work when you are required and for you it will be business as usual.

In the medical profession there is no work from home concept which has recently become very popular since the COVID pandemic.

You may have realized and seen that during the lockdown during the pandemic everybody was advised by the authorities to stay at home and not to leave their house but doctors not only have to leave their house but have to go to work at the hospital. The hospitals became overburdened and extremely busy so the doctors and nurses became so busy at work that sometime they have to even skip their meals to look after the sick patients and they have to stay back for extra hours during their shifts

As doctors are also human beings lots of them also sadly succumbed to this nasty and deadly virus and as per the WHO (World Health Organization) recommendations even if they were not very unwell they were not allowed to come to the hospital for the fear of them spreading it to their healthier patients so ultimately the working man power went down to the extent that they were fewer doctors looking after more number of sick patients.

To cope with this extraordinary situation extraordinary measures have to be taken which meant doctors from different specialties were roped in to help their colleagues for example Pediatricians looking after adult patients with the help and supervision of the adult physician colleagues.

And as the pandemic lingered on the doctor started to have mental and physical fatigue and started to have burnout. But in spite of all that, most doctors felt that working during a pandemic was the most satisfying part of their career and the biggest service they could do humbly to mankind. The general public and people across the word in return appreciated whole heartedly the hard work and sacrifices doctors made during this extraordinary period by coming out at their balconies of their houses and clapping for health care professionals and this you must have seen on your television screens quite a few times.

Doctors made lots of sacrifices during their working during the pandemic as lots of them will not even come home and will sleep in the hospital accommodation so that they do not expose their families to this deadly virus. Except people working in healthcare like doctors and nurses I can't think of any other profession where people have to make so many sacrifices to help others

CHAPTER 4

THE WHITE COAT CHRONICLES: EMBRACING THE JOURNEY OF CHALLENGES AND SACRIFICES IN MEDICINE

"Becoming a doctor means embracing a lifelong journey of learning, compassion, and healing."

What it will mean to you when you qualify as a doctor especially if you come from the countries like India, China, Africa or South America that you may have to take care of lots of patients and you may be the only doctor available in the radius of hundreds of miles and you may also not have best of the infrastructure and health care facilities to treat these patients.

You have to completely rely on your clinical skills to make a quick decision like a pilot of the fighter jet plane, to save the life of a patient as you may not have any doctor colleague or a senior or a junior who may guide or help you in making those critical decisions.

But if you are deciding to choose medicine as a career because you want to serve the society and especially the deprived population of your country you will get the best career satisfaction while working in these remote areas. You may not become rich with money but the respect and the popularity you will gain within the local community will be unparalleled and doctors in these areas are treated like superheroes by the local population which will be indebted forever for your services.

I would like to share my personal perspective and experience in this context. My father was a General physician in India where I grew up as a child. He was working in the government run Primary Health Care Centers which are in rural and remote areas. He was a very honest and dedicated doctor so he would go and work in any part of the state where the government would ask him to go and as a child I had to follow him whenever he was posted. I still have the memory of him working in a very remote village where he was the only doctor where there was no electricity at all so sometimes we would sit under the tree to see the patients and our house was only 100 meters away from this small hospital. He would be on call 24/7 which means the patients will come to see him at any time. My father will see these patients and then after giving the primary care if needed he would ask them to go to secondary level hospital in a city but most of these villages were so poor they could not afford lots of time to have the transport to travel and reach those secondary care hospitals and they may even sadly die. After serving in this village for about 6 years he was then posted to a state called Uttarakhand which is where the Himalayas are. So we used to live in these mountains and he would go by foot walking to his hospital which was a relatively bigger hospital than his previous hospital in the village as there were about 4- 5 doctors.

My father was a very good clinician and I say that because even as a child I have lots of memories of people flocking to see him and treating him like a God. As my father will not take any money in return to his service they will bring vegetables and fruits from their own farms. When he left these places I saw lots of people coming to meet him and crying as they did not want him to leave because they did not see a doctor like him before.

The reason for that was and still is that most doctors who are employed by the government do not want to go to these remote places even if they go they will ask money in return for their services from these poor villagers.

> "In medicine, every patient is an opportunity to touch someone's life and bring hope and healing."

One other thing to keep in mind is that when as the doctor you are serving these deprived areas your family has to make sacrifices. As a child, to go to a decent School I had to travel miles with public transport or in the hilly areas by foot and that I am talking about from the age of 4 to 12.

No wonder why doctors do not want to serve these remote areas and lots of responsibility lies with the local government to provide decent schools and basic infrastructure to these doctors and their families because there is no other profession I can think of where people have to be posted and work and most importantly be physically present in those villages.

Working of the doctors in day to day life no

matter which specialty you are in whether you are an Emergency physician, a Neurosurgeon or a General physician is not as exciting, adventurous and glamorous as the character of Dr Gregory House in the House or George Clooney as Doug Ross in ER or Doctor Meredith Grey in Grey's Anatomy, some of the most popular American medical drama TV series.

Quite understandably the directors and the producers of any TV drama series have to dramatize the working of their characters which happen to be all doctors in these series, to keep the audience engaged and all of these did their job very well in that respect as they were the most popular TV drama series. I think in a way these TV shows do give the impression to the public that a doctor's life in and out of the hospital is not as boring as they might think.

As lots of people thankfully do not visit emergency department or hospital frequently and perhaps meet the doctors for few minutes or hours in the emergency department and do not even know that this particular doctor is doing 12 or 24 hour shift and how busy he or she has been managing patients during their shifts

To give them some credit I think these kind of TV drama series may encourage young people like you to join the medicine and become one of those characters, however this might be like deciding to join Army after playing the video game Call of Duty

In real life working as a doctor may not be as

glamorous as shown in any TV drama series or in the films. Although the working routine will vary from one specialty to another, on a daily basis doctors will see a patient in the clinic in what we call an outpatient setting.

CHAPTER 5

BEYOND THE WHITE COAT: UNVEILING THE EXTRAORDINARY JOURNEY OF MEDICINE'S HEROES

"Choosing medicine is a commitment to a lifetime of growth, perseverance, and making a positive impact on society."

Y ou can as a doctor become famous for work in fields outside of medicine.

I'll give you some examples.

Dr Mae Jemison went into orbit aboard the Space Shuttle Endeavour in 1992 and became the first African American woman in space. She is also a trained medical doctor, served as a Medical Officer in the Peace Corps and currently runs BioSentient Corp, a medical technology company.

Dr. Ben Carson, well known face in American politics, is an retired neurosurgeon, academic, author, and politician who served as the 17th United States Secretary of Housing and Urban Development and he was a candidate for President of the United States in the 2016 Republican primaries. Dr Carson became the director of pediatric neurosurgery at the Johns Hopkins Children's Center in 1984 at age 33, then the youngest chief of pediatric neurosurgery in the United States.

Dr. Henry Heimlich, a thoracic surgeon who invented the Heimlich maneuver, a technique for dislodging food or other objects from a choking person's airway. This technique is taught in all the life support courses to the doctors around the world and has saved thousands of lives so far. Not only that, his other big contribution in the field of medicine is that he invented the chest drainage flutter valve (also called the Heimlich valve). The design of the valve allows air and blood to drain from the chest cavity in order to allow a collapsed lung to re-expand. The invention was credited with saving the lives of hundreds of American soldiers in the Vietnam War

Dr. Oliver Sacks, a neurologist and author who wrote popular books on neuroscience and case studies of neurological disorders, including "Awakenings" which was adapted into an Academy Award-nominated feature film in1990, starring Robin Williams and Robert De Niro.

Dr. Sanjay Gupta, a well known face in American TV, was the host of the CNN show Sanjay Gupta MD for which he has won multiple Emmy Awards. He is a neurosurgeon and medical correspondent for CNN.

Dr. Atul Gawande, a surgeon and writer who has written several best-selling books on healthcare, including "Being Mortal" and "The Checklist Manifesto". In 2020, he was named a member of President-elect Joe Biden's COVID-19 Advisory Board.

When Doctors Take Center Stage In Cinema

There are some doctors who have chosen to pursue careers in the film industry. Here are some examples:

Dr. Ken Jeong is a comedian and actor who is best known for his roles in movies such as "The Hangover" and TV shows like "Community". He was a practicing physician before transitioning to comedy and acting.

George Miller is an Australian filmmaker and former medical doctor. He earned his medical degree from the University of New South Wales and worked as a doctor in Sydney for a few years before transitioning to a career in film. He is best known for his work as the director and co-writer of the Mad Max film series, which were all big hits.

CHAPTER 6

THE HEALING HANDS CENSUS: ILLUMINATING THE ENIGMATIC WORLD OF THE DOCTORS' WORKFORCE

According to the World Health Organization (WHO), as of 2020, approximately 70% of the global health workforce is made up of women, and this proportion has been increasing in recent years. However, the proportion of female medical students varies widely by country and region.

Using a career in medicine has distinct advantages as compared to other professions. You have job security as no matter which country your planning to study and practice medicine there will not be any shortage of jobs in Healthcare profession

The study, titled "Measuring the availability of human resources for health and its relationship to universal health coverage for 204 countries and territories from 1990 to 2019: A Systematic analysis for the Global Burden of Disease Study 2019," was published in May 2023 by The Lancet, a well known medical journal.

According to this study, globally, as of 2019, the world had 104 million health workers, including 12.8 million physicians. In total, the 2019 national health workforces fell short of 6·4 million physicians.

For physicians, the global density was estimated to 16.7 per 10,000 population. Densities ranged from 2.9 physicians for every 10,000 people in sub-Saharan Africa to 38.3 per 10,000 in Central Europe, Eastern Europe, and Central Asia. Cuba also stood out, with a density of 84.4 per 10,000 compared to 2.1 in Haiti.

According to this study Cuba has almost 50,000 medical professors, more than 100,000 doctors and around 100,000 nurses. With an average of 9 doctors and 9 nurses per 1,000 inhabitants, Cuba is today one of the best equipped nations in the world in this sector.

There is something called doctor patient ratio, where

you look at the data of number of working doctors per 1000 inhabitants and higher the number of doctors is, it indirectly means better healthcare.

If we look at the data provided by Organization for Economic Co-operation and Development (OECD) data from 2021, which is the most updated data, in two of the most populated countries which is China and India the ratio is 1-2 doctor per 1000 people which is one of the lowest as compared to 5 doctor per 1000 population, which is highest. You may be surprised to know that countries with very advanced health care like the USA, UK and Canada are actually quite low in the list of countries with an average of only 3 doctors per 1000 people. Austria is on top of that list with 5.2 doctors per 1,000 inhabitants.

So what these data suggest is that we will of course need more and more doctors in coming years, however you need to understand that this is a global data and as mentioned in the study the demand varies from one country to another and one region to another.

But when we look at these data, we have to keep in mind particularly in countries like India and China where there is a lot of wealth disparity that this ratio can vary hugely and in remote villages and small towns there may not be even one qualified doctor for thousands of patients.

CHAPTER 7

EMBRACING AUTONOMY: UNVEILING THE THRILLING JOURNEY OF WORKING FOR YOURSELF OR WORKING FOR OTHERS

"You have within you right now, everything you need to conquer the

world." - The Karate Kid

You can either discover the joys and triumphs of building your own empire, where you become the architect of your destiny, navigating uncharted territories, and reaping the rewards of your dedication and ingenuity.

On the other side lies the realm of working for someone else, a captivating landscape where collaboration, stability, and structured growth become the foundation of success.

If you are planning to settle down in big urban cities then you will have more competition as there will be more people applying for fewer jobs available. This will be the case across all specialties. It also depends of course in which country you are graduating from and intending to settle down and practice.

Overall you will not have to struggle to get the job or even establish your own private practice by opening a clinic of your own. You can get attached to a hospital to perform your operations and use their operating theaters if you are surgeon and if you're a physician and want to manage your patient as an in-patient if they require the care which cannot be provided in outpatient settings for example giving fluids, antibiotics etc. then you can also be attached to a hospital.

One good thing about being a doctor is that you do not have to work for an employer and you can easily work for yourself as long as you are registered with the local medical registration governing bodies and you comply with the strict regulatory guidelines to maintain your medical professional license.

There are of course pros and cons of working on your own as an individual or working with your other doctor colleagues who can all come together and open up a medical center. Again depending on the country which you are planning to practice the regulations vary, however in most countries you should be able to establish either on your own or with other doctors and health care professionals such as the nurses and therapists like physiotherapist or occupational therapist.

If you are going to run your own clinic and your own practice you have to hire a manager to run that facility. Advantages of running your own clinical practice or your own hospital is that you are the boss of your own practice. You can run that as a business and can provide a very high quality service to your patients.

But if you are going to run your own hospital or clinic, you should be good in managing the finances in which most doctors are not good at, however the new generation of doctors like yourself are more astute and financially savvy as compared to the doctors of my generation so that may not be a problem.

The success of this venture like any other business will depend on the country you are going to open it and the location in that particular country whether it's urban or rural. You may have to work really hard spending lots of hours in your own facility. If you are a newly qualified specialist the patients of that area may not know you and it may take a few years for you to establish and gain the confidence of the patients so that they can trust you and keep coming back to see you as a doctor which may take your time away from your family as you will be inclined to spend more time at work at your own clinic or hospital.

My personal experience in opening up my own private clinic for children and babies soon after specializing and finishing my training in pediatrics and newborns has not been very good for various reasons. Most important one was that I started it when I was very young and had no knowledge and experience of how to run a business as a doctor, only thing I thought I was good at that time was looking after children's and newborns as I had my training from one of the top institutes in India and did one year further fellowship at a big tertiary hospital in the capital of India.

I was full of confidence and had kind of wrong thinking that it is better to start your own practice when you are young and ventured into that in a completely new city where patients and people did not knew me at all and I had to compete with so many other pediatricians who were already established and had years of practice under their belt. Having said that, it did not take me very long to establish my own practice because of the high quality training I had. I was fortunate enough to get trained under the supervision of the professors who were not only good academicians but also very good mentors and trainers.

After practicing alone for four years I did not see myself progressing in my career apart from earning a little bit of money and most importantly I was unable to spend time with my parents, my wife and my little kid, so eventually I closed that clinic, sold everything off and went to England.

So if you ask me, my personal advice would be even if you're planning to open your own set up please do not do that until after few years of your training and try to spend time learning new things and procedures and best way to do that is to work in a established hospital where you have fixed hours of working so that you can spend time with your family and friends which is really important when you are young.

I did not understand the important fact that this time would never come back again and that my professional career can wait for a few years. Starting any new business is an adventure which takes away lots of your precious moments which never come back again.

You also have to deal with buying or renting the

building where you are going to open this facility and you have to invest in buying sophisticated equipment which is getting more and more expensive nowadays. Not only that, they get irrelevant after a few years like any other technology like your mobile phone, laptop or any other kind of software.

Even if you do not buy any expensive equipment and want to practice just like a family physician, you still have to invest in an electronic health record which is a software produced by lots of companies mostly based in the USA, as now keeping the medical records on paper is becoming obsolete in most countries. All the medical health records now are going paperless..

If you are planning to open a hospital then of course it is a big investment and you may also need a financier or take out a big loan to finance your project.

There is a trend nowadays that lots of doctors of different or same specialties are coming together to open multi-specialty outpatient clinics and a Day Care Centre where the patients get elective not so complex surgeries and procedures done. They can be discharged home on the same day of surgery.

Opening a facility with other doctors, I think is a very good option, however it requires all the doctors collaborating in this project and to have the same kind of mindset and commitment to provide high quality patient care and keep patient care before the finances and profitability.

I have seen personally that these kinds of joint ventures either close or split up into smaller units because of the personality clashes between the doctors who initially try to work together.

As far as working in a hospital whether it's a government or private and doing a salaried job is concerned there would be lots of options and opportunities depending on which country you are going to work and whether you're going to work in a bigger city or remote areas.

If you are going to work in a private hospital lots of hospitals are giving this option of either working full time for them and they will pay you a fixed salary or you can earn based on the number of patients you see in outpatient clinics or admit and do any kind of surgical procedures.

Out of all those options, which one you choose will depend on whether you are already established in the community as a respected and a popular doctor thus you have a good patient base and in that case you can work more or less independently without the hassle of supervising and doing the administrative work which will help you to concentrate more on your clinical work.

However the downside will be, its again like running your own practice where your revenue and earnings may go up and down depending on how many holidays you take per year and quite importantly if the competition around your hospital is increasing in your particular specialty and locality, which may give patients more choices in choosing different hospitals, maybe because of the better insurance cover or simply because they have more five star kind of facility of which patients nowadays are demanding and looking for.

Patients now a day do not want to compromise in the quality of care they get not only from clinical point of view but also they are looking for other factors such as the cleanliness of the hospital, the food they get served, the attitude of the people working in that hospital such as the administrative staff and the nurses and so forth. All these factors will be beyond your control as a doctor as you do not own this hospital and management of that hospital will run it the way they think is best.

If you work for a private hospital on a fixed salary then you don't have to worry about your earnings per month whether you go on holiday or not, whether you see fewer patients and whether the competition around that hospital has increased or not. None of these factors should affect you, which means you will have more time to spend with your family and you can do more leisure activities and look after your health as well, which unfortunately and ironically is the last priority doctors have for themselves.

If you work for a government hospital for example I was working for National Health Services in UK which

I have to say is one of the best health care system in the world at its free for the public and patients at the point of contact which means the people living in Britain do not pay any Health Care Insurance or to the doctor or hospital when they visit emergency department of the hospital or even when they see a General Physician or a Specialist for their treatment whether it's for the cancer or the heart problem or diabetes.

Not only that, they also get medications with a very subsidized rate of fixed prescription charges which at the time of writing is around 10 British Pounds, no matter how much is the real cost of the medication in that prescription. It could be hundreds or thousands of British pounds. In case even if any patient needs surgery of any kind whether it's a brain surgery or a heart surgery patient does not pay a single penny if they are legitimately living and working in the UK.

The National Health Services in the United Kingdom is all funded by the government by taxpayers money.

Similarly countries like Sweden, Norway, Finland, Belgium, Netherlands, Canada and Japan have one of the best Public Health systems in the world.

There are countries like China and India, the two of the world's most populous countries, which also have Public Health systems which are free to the public and funded by the government but the quality of health care provided is inconsistent and varies a lot between urban and rural areas. So ultimately in these countries the citizens and the residents who can afford to pay opt for private medical care.

The health care system in the United States of America, which is the richest country in the world ironically does not have Universal Healthcare.

The US government does not provide Health benefits to the citizens or the residents so any time you get medical care someone has to pay for it. It could be your Health Insurance or you will be paying from your own pocket.

Report published by the Commonwealth fund in 2021 which compared the Performance of the Healthcare Systems of the 11 High income countries of the United States ranked last despite spending a substantially large amount of GDP on Healthcare.

So in summary whether you work independently and run your own clinic or hospital or you work as an employee for a government or a privately run Hospital will all depend on your preferences and your choices which you will make to balance your professional career and your personal lifestyle and most importantly your commitment to the family time.

These are not easy decisions to make especially when you are young and you have just come out in the field after finishing your training as a fresh and new specialist doctor.

Lots of time our circumstances dictate and compel us

to make tough decisions in our life and this might be one of those but whatever you decide, that will not be end of the word and you can always switch from one pathway to another without much of a problem. I have seen this happening lots of time in my professional career to my other professional colleagues and I myself has done this several times and in doing so even moved from one country to another.

CHAPTER 8

UNVEILING THE MEDICAL FRONTIER: THE EXTRAORDINARY JOURNEY OF RESEARCH IN MEDICINE

"Medicine offers endless opportunities for innovation, research, and making groundbreaking discoveries that can change lives."

When you enter medical school and finally qualify as a doctor you have two pathways to choose. You can go either in clinical medicine and treat the patients or you can go into Medical Research. It depends in which country you are going to study and qualify as a doctor when choose Medical Research as the career as it requires lots of funding and if you are going to be the part of the research team who is developing a new drug to treat medical conditions then you should be aware that most of these researches are funded by Pharmaceutical companies.

And remember it may take years and years from starting to develop this drug into the laboratory to finally reaching the patients for the treatment and not all the drugs successfully reach that final stage. Your job mostly will be to conduct and supervise the trials called Phase 2 and Phase 3 trial of these drug or new form of treatment in the healthy volunteers and then in patients

Similarly you can also conduct or join the research projects where new forms of non-pharmacological treatment are being tested in the patients most of these are called randomized control trials where two forms of treatments are available but we don't know which one is better for the patients and you can be initially as a fresh post graduate medical student be part of these trials being supervised by your supervisor who generally are the professors in medicine and you can even work towards getting PhD degree which is in addition to your post graduate degree which varies from one country to another for example in North America and India it's called MD and in UK it's MRCP (Member of Royal College of Physicians) or MRCS (Member of Royal College of Surgeons) or in Germany PG Medical Program.

The duration of these clinical Research trials may vary from one to ten years depending on effectiveness of what kind of treatment, medical or surgical you are investigating for. Lots of time these trials are done not only to look for effectiveness but also to see that they are not causing any harm to the patients which is the basic philosophy and principle of medicine that whatever you do to the patients, even if you cannot make the patient better at least don't do any harm.

If you are interested in doing research in medicine and aiming to develop some break through diagnostic tests or the treatment which may transform the lives of the patients and will significantly reduce the morbidity or mortality of the patients then by choosing medicine as a career you will be doing a great service to wider section of society as millions of people across the word will be directly benefiting from your research which will be across the boundaries of the Nations and different strata of the society whether they are rich or poor they will all be benefited equally.

There Are Thousands Of Examples Of The Breakthrough Research Done By The Doctors.

I will mention here a few of them, whom most of you must be familiar with.

Dr. Jonas Salk, an American physician and medical researcher, developed the first successful polio vaccine. His work helped eradicate polio as a widespread disease and saved countless lives.

Dr. Alexander Fleming was a Scottish physician and microbiologist who discovered penicillin, the first antibiotic. His discovery revolutionized the treatment of bacterial infections and laid the foundation for the development of numerous other antibiotics.

Dr. Robert Koch, a German physician, is considered one of the founders of modern bacteriology. He identified the causative agents for several diseases, including tuberculosis, cholera, and anthrax. His work laid the foundation for the field of medical microbiology and contributed significantly to our understanding of infectious diseases.

If you are thinking of going into medicine because you want to be a top researcher in the field of medicine remember that the top quality research laboratories require lot of funding and is mostly done in resource rich countries and you also need to find a mentor who will guide you through the initial part of your research project and your guide will be the one who will help you to write a research project to get the right funding.

You need to bear in mind that any other research project might take years and years until you achieve the goals and objectives of your research and you may not get to the end point where you want to be which might be frustrating for you and your team.

So you have to have that kind of personality which is very inquisitive, you should have lots of patience and you are committed and dedicated to do research which is based in the laboratory where you will not have any interaction with the patients, If you are happy with this kind of professional life then yes of course by all means choose medicine as a career to become full time medical researcher.

There are lots of doctors who also do clinical trials and are either hired by the pharmaceutical industry to do what is known in the industry as phase 2 and phase 3 trials. It is mandatory by law and the regulatory authorities of all countries that before launching a new drug in the market to be used by the public and the patients these different phases of trials are done.

The purpose of the trials is to know first of all that these drugs are safe to be used in humans and are not causing any harm and secondly they have proven efficacy as compared to placebo which could be just a water or non-reactive salt. As during the trials the two groups of patients are blindly treated either with the medication which is being tested or given a placebo; these are called double blind trials, which means neither the researcher nor the participant knows which treatment they are receiving until the clinical trial is over and the data is analyzed.

You can work for these pharmaceutical companies as a clinical drug trial researcher but again remember in this kind of job you will not be seeing the patients in a traditional sense however the patience under the drug trial will be your responsibility as a doctor and you will be examining them and monitoring their vital signs.

Apart from working for pharmaceutical companies to do clinical trials lots of doctors and clinicians do randomized control trials on the patients admitted to the hospitals where they are comparing to different modes of treatment both of which are safe and have been approved to be used by the relevant health authorities but as a doctor we just want to know which one is more effective than other.

To conduct these kinds of randomized trials within the hospital settings the principal investigator or researcher has to go through different steps of approval from the committee in the hospital which regulates every research project. These are known as Research and ethics committee.

A research and ethics committee is a group of

people appointed to review research proposals to assess formally if the research is ethical. This means the research must conform to recognized ethical standards, which includes respecting the dignity, rights, safety and well-being of the people who take part.

If you are interested in doing research and clinical trials along with your usual clinical work you can do that provided you are working in an academic institute or a big government or private run Hospital.

Conducting these trials requires a research set of mind which means you are inquisitive and curious to know which kind of treatment mode will be better for the patients. You have to keep some time out of your busy clinical schedule to spend in conducting these trials, which are usually done as a team so you may be part of a team which includes other healthcare professionals as well.

If you have conducted a high quality clinical trial you and your team can submit this to reputed international journals for publication and by doing this you will be helping and disseminating very useful outcomes of your trial to your other medical colleagues across the word which may help them change the way they practice to manage their patients.

There are lots and lots of interesting examples of such trials done across the word which have completely transformed and improved the outcome of the patients.

In the 1960s two British doctors in Liverpool UK, Richard Smithells a Pediatrician and Elizabeth Hibbard, a Obstetrician did a multi-center Intervention study which means it was done across many hospitals

Participants of this trial were the women in their early pregnancy.

This was the randomized control trial which means the participants were divided into two groups one group was given vitamin called Folic acid and the other group not supplemented with this vitamin and they found that the group of women's who were supplemented with Folic acid had significantly less chances of their babies developing serious birth defects, most notably a defect where the spine of the baby is not fully formed which can lead to paralysis of the legs and even the death.

Since the result of this trial was published all the pregnant women in the early pregnancy or the women who are planning to become pregnant are given Folic acid on a daily basis as a vitamin supplement and this has significantly reduced the chances of their baby getting spinal malformations.

Not only that, 60 countries including the United States of America have started the policy of mandatory fortification of flour with Folic acid.

So you can see how such a simple intervention

has significantly reduced the morbidity in newborn babies.it just needed a scientific thinking and inquisitiveness from the two doctors.

So While you are taking care of your patients on a day to day basis at the same time you can also conduct research trials and Improve the quality of health of a bigger population as the outcome of your research trial will have wider applicability and will not be restricted to one geographical area.

Doing research is one of the ways to reach out to the society, gain popularity and be known worldwide, however for most researchers the ultimate aim is to improve quality of health and reduce the morbidity and mortality of every world citizen.

CHAPTER 9

HEALING HEROES:
UNMASKING
THE VITAL ROLE
OF DOCTORS -
ILLUMINATING
THE
EXTRAORDINARY
IMPACT OF
MEDICAL
MARVELS ON
SOCIETY

"Heroes are made by the paths they choose, not the powers they are graced with." - Iron Man

There are lots of examples of doctors who with their background knowledge in medicine have helped particularly economically deprived and socially alienated section of the society either by forming and leading a charity organization, being part or the head of the government organizations and advising the government how to improve the quality of health of their citizens or by writing books on different healthcare issues and suggesting solutions for them.

These examples are not only from resource rich countries like the United States of America but also from Somalia, one of the poorest countries in the world.

Dr. Devi Shetty is an Indian cardiac surgeon and entrepreneur. He is the founder of Narayana Health, a healthcare group that provides high-quality and affordable medical services. Dr. Shetty has been recognized for his innovative approaches to cardiac surgery and for making healthcare more accessible to people in India and other developing countries.

Dr. Denis Mukwege is a Congolese gynecologist and human rights activist. He is known for his work in providing surgical care to women who have experienced sexual violence in the Democratic Republic of Congo. Dr. Mukwege has received international recognition for his efforts to address the physical and psychological impact of sexual violence and to advocate for the rights of survivors.

Dr. Hawa Abdi was a Somali physician and human rights activist who dedicated her career to providing healthcare and humanitarian assistance to people affected by conflict in Somalia. She established the Dr. Hawa Abdi Foundation, which operated a hospital and a camp for internally displaced persons. Dr. Abdi's work in providing medical care and advocating for women's rights earned her numerous accolades and global recognition.

Dr. Catherine Hamlin, an Australian obstetrician and gynecologist, dedicated her life to treating obstetric fistula, a devastating childbirth injury, in Ethiopia. She co-founded the Hamlin Fistula Hospital, where thousands of women have received life-changing surgical care. Dr. Hamlin's work has transformed the lives of countless women and brought global attention to the issue of obstetric fistula.

CHAPTER 10

CAREER CROSSROADS: NAVIGATING THE MAZE OF POSSIBILITIES AND OTHER OPTIONS AVAILABLE

"Choose a job you love, and you will never have to work a day in your life." - The Pursuit of Happyness

Although it's very hard and time consuming for me to compare so many other career choices which you as a High School or Higher Secondary student may have nowadays as compared to in the 80s and 90s when we were only left with two or three options.

I would like to discuss and compare three other top professions which most of you might be considering other than medicine. These are computer sciences, Law and career in finance or business industry.

For each of these I will make comparisons in four sub headings which are Education, Job stability, Work life balance and Job satisfaction

I have already discussed these four aspects in reference to medicine as a career in great detail, so not going to repeat that again here.

Coding Your Destiny: Embark on an Exciting Journey in Pursuit of a Career in Computer Science

Computer science typically requires a bachelor's degree in computer engineering or a related field which is for three to four years duration depending on in which country you are going to study. Then after finishing bachelor's degree, depending on the specialization some roles may require additional certifications or advanced degrees such as a Masters which is typically for one to two years and it provides you with a more specialized set of skills such as Artificial Intelligence which is new kid on the block.

As far as Job Stability is concerned, the field of computer engineering is in high demand and will remain in demand for an infinite number of years as our dependence on computers is increasing day by day, and this dependence on computers is not only in work life but also in our personal day to day life.

With time there will be a growing need for professionals in areas such as software development, cybersecurity, and artificial intelligence. So overall job stability can be relatively strong in this field.

Computer engineering careers can offer good work-life balance, with opportunities for flexible working hours and remote work, which became so popular during COVID-19 pandemic. Although this was a necessity during those difficult times, now even during the post COVID era most computer professionals are not willing to give up remote working and opting for hybrid models which even the employers are agreeing with.

So now the world has learned the new model of working which is work from home and this is I have to say one of the positive outcomes of the COVID-19 pandemic. It has certainly improved the work life balance of computer professionals and lots of other such professionals, whose job requirements give them this option of working to choose.

However, project deadlines or challenging projects require additional hours or overtime.

Computer engineers often find satisfaction in solving complex problems, developing innovative technologies, and being at the forefront of technological advancements. They can work in diverse industries and contribute to shaping the future through technology.

Dollars or Dreams: Deciphering Your Financial Destiny - Unraveling the Enigmatic Journey of Pursuing a Career in Finance

Career in finance can start with a bachelor's degree in finance, economics, or a related field. Advanced degrees, such as an MBA or a master's in finance, can enhance your career prospects.

As far as job stability is concerned the finance industry offers a range of roles, including financial analysis, investment banking, financial planning, and risk management. While job stability can vary depending on economic conditions and industry changes, finance professionals are generally in great demand.

Work-life balance in finance can vary depending on the specific role and company culture. Certain positions, such as investment banking, may involve long hours and high-pressure environments, for example Investment bankers and Hedge fund managers working in London City or Financial District of New York work very long hours but they are financially rewarding while other roles offer more predictable schedules.

Finance professionals often find satisfaction in analyzing financial data, making strategic decisions, and helping individuals or businesses achieve their financial goals. The industry offers opportunities for career growth and potential for high earnings.

Delving into the Intriguing Dilemma of Becoming a Lawyer or Attorney

Career in Law like Medicine in countries like the USA and lots of European countries requires a longer period of studies, and go through aptitude tests and entrance exams.

A legal career typically requires a bachelor's degree followed by a Juris Doctor (JD) degree from an accredited law school in the USA, so it takes at least seven years to graduate as Attorney. In UK they are called Solicitors and it takes about six to seven years before they can practice Law

In most countries they have to pass exams like the Bar exam in the USA or equivalent to that in the UK and Europe before they can practice Law.

The overall timeline to become a lawyer in Europe can range from five to seven years or longer, depending on the country.

Similarly the total duration to become a Lawyer in India, including the LLB program, enrollment with the Bar Council, apprenticeship, and passing the bar examination, generally takes around five to six years.

The legal profession can provide job stability, especially in established law firms or government agencies. However, competition for certain positions can be intense, and the job market can be influenced by economic factors.

Work-life balance in law can be challenging like in medicine, particularly in the early stages of a legal career. Lawyers often work long hours, handle heavy workloads, and face strict deadlines. However, as professionals advance in their careers, they may gain more control over their schedules.

According to an American Bar Association survey conducted in 2019, around 64% of lawyers in the United States reported being somewhat or very satisfied with their careers, which is more than 50% and its as good as in any other profession.

Lawyers have the opportunity to advocate for justice, help clients navigate legal issues, and make a positive impact in society. They can specialize in various areas of law.

CHAPTER 11

UNLEASHING YOUR INNER SUPER DOC: THE EPIC JOURNEY OF LIFELONG LEARNING AND GROWTH THROUGH CONTINUOUS PROFESSIONAL DEVELOPMENT

A career in medicine requires commitment to life-long learning in order to remain fit to practice and provide the best possible care to your patients.

Medicine is one of the few professions in which until you completely retire you have to keep updating your knowledge and skills to keep your professional license active. So basically you remain a student throughout your professional career. Your learning doesn't stop after graduation or post-graduation. And moreover this is not optional you have to continuously keep updating yourself and learning and submit the proof of that to your governing licensing authorities.

All the doctors and in fact all the health care professionals have to do something called continuous professional development (CPD) which includes any informal or formal learning activities and training during their active career.

There are lots of good reasons to do CPD. Doctors need to keep up to date with the latest guidelines and regulations. This will help them to maintain their fitness to practice and strengthen the quality of care and safety they give to patients.

Some components are mandatory for example these are called Life support courses and you may have heard about basic life support (BLS), which now lots of High Schools are doing for their students. By doing these courses students learn how to recognize Life threatening emergencies which can happen in a shopping mall, on a street or even at home to any of your family members. If you are BLS trained you can provide CPR which is cardiopulmonary resuscitation to the victims, a classic example being a person choking with the food in a restaurant.

Doctors are typically required to track and report their CPD activities to the relevant regulatory bodies to demonstrate compliance with CPD requirements to keep their Professional License active. Failure to meet CPD obligations may result in penalties or the restriction of a Doctor's ability to practice medicine.

CPD requirements can include attending seminars, workshops, webinars, conferences, or participating in online courses, mentoring programs, or writing and publications in listed medical journals.

CHAPTER 12

DIAGNOSIS IN THE DIGITAL AGE: UNRAVELING THE INTRIGUING DR GOOGLE PHENOMENON

In our medical fraternity there is something called the "Dr. Google" phenomenon, which has been a buzzword for quite some time. You may or may not be aware of this but basically the "Dr. Google" phenomenon refers to the tendency of patients to turn to the internet, search engines, and online sources for health information and self-diagnosis.

I am pretty sure all of you, as you are tech savvy

generation must be relying on internet search engines such as Google or now the new phenomenon, chat GPT, which is increasingly becoming more popular.

As a doctor I completely agree that by using online information patients feel more empowered and better informed about their health.

However one of the downsides of the internet is the abundance of inaccurate or unreliable health information. Patients then end up having conflicting or misleading information, which as a consequence leads to unnecessary anxiety, self-diagnosis, or incorrect assumptions about their health condition.

This then can create challenges for doctors who need to address and correct misconceptions during consultations.

Not only that, the worst thing is that the "Dr. Google" approach can often undermine trust in the doctor-patient relationship. The trust between the doctor and patient has always been the fundamental basis of good doctor patient relationship and when patients start to question or challenge the doctor's expertise based on information they found online, the trust factor is broken which eventually may breakdown doctor patient relationship, which then leads to patients doing doctor shopping, means hopping from one doctor clinic hospital to another one, which may delay their diagnosis and treatment, which is real and present danger.

Myself and all my doctors colleagues are facing problems with this "Dr. Google" phenomenon. Almost every patient, even in life threatening and serious conditions, worryingly challenges the doctor's decision, which may delay the right treatment and consequently the overall outcome of that patient.

I think you guys have an edge over the doctors of my generation when dealing with these patients, who think Dr Google can treat their medical conditions. They think either they don't need to go to a doctors clinic to seek medical advice or they can tell the doctors how their illness should be managed.

As a doctor now we are also learning the tricks to handle these patients. One thing most doctors do or at least I do is that I Google myself common health conditions in children and see what information I get from the internet. This at least prepares me to answer queries of parents in a better way. Also it helps me to direct and navigate them to the right and legitimate websites which give scientific and evidence based information and advice to the public.

Thankfully there are lots of health organizations which are providing patient information leaflets in simple layman's terminology about different health conditions. For example in the UK they can go to the NHS website or for the common health conditions. For children, American Academy of Pediatrics or Royal College of Pediatrics and child health are very good sites for them to read about common childhood health issues including vaccines and immunization . You may not believe it, but there are lots of parents who are misguided by anti-vaccine groups, which are very active on the internet and these legitimate websites try to clear myths and misconceptions surrounding vaccines. Also various hospitals across the world have the information for the public to read on common health issues.

Our job as healthcare professionals is first to read these leaflets ourselves and be convinced that information given is correct, before suggesting the patients to go to those websites so that after reading if they have any questions or queries we are better prepared to answer those.

In my opinion, the medical schools now should start Including in their curriculum, teaching medical students how to get better and deal with the information available on the internet to the public and how to respond as a doctor when faced with the patients who come loaded with that information which may or may not be correct.

As we are living in the world of information technology and nowadays we are talking about artificial intelligence making the diagnosis, it's high time that doctors also get used to familiarizing themselves with these technological advances.

Recently, just out of interest I tried putting the symptoms of a child on chat GPT, to see what diagnosis it comes up with after putting some symptoms. What I found was reassuring that although it is giving a list of diagnoses and not just one but most reassuringly, it always says that you must consult a doctor. It does help me though, as by knowing what differential diagnosis it has suggested, I am prepared that the patient is going to ask me in the clinic about those diagnoses, which will help me in handling those questions better.

It is interesting how different doctors are handling these patients. One of my colleagues told me that after listening to the patient all about what the internet has told them he politely asks them - can I please now take over from Dr Google !!

It is essential for doctors to acknowledge and address patients' concerns while providing evidence-based information to maintain trust and credibility.

CHAPTER 13

THE GREAT PAUSE: EXPLORING THE TRUTH BEHIND TAKING A CAREER BREAK IN MEDICINE

"Life's too short to be stuck in a job you don't love. It's time to take a leap and find what makes you happy." - Yes Man

S tep into the world of medical professionals, where the notion of taking a career break is often shrouded in mystery and uncertainty.

At some point in your career in medicine as a doctor you might like to take a career break and do something which you always dreamed of and enjoy doing but never had time because of your demanding work schedule.

For example you may have an innovative idea about a health related start-up or you want to develop and design an App for mobile devices. You may have a brilliant idea about developing such an App or developing tech solutions in health as a doctor and now is the time you think is right for you to do so. But to do so, you will need a lot of time and effort which may not be possible while you are full time as a doctor.

You might be a gifted musician and now you want to take your passion for music further by creating brilliant compositions, or you might like to be part of a musical band and do live performances.

Or like me who has still not given up the idea of directing at least a short film. You might like to take a career break and do a diploma course in filmmaking from the New York film academy. Who knows you may be the next George Miller, an Australian filmmaker and former medical doctor who directed and co-wrote a very successful franchise of Mad Max movies.

So to convert your dreams into reality you will need time off and a career break from the medicine for a certain period of time which may vary from a few months to a couple of years.

Now this is the tricky bit as in medicine to practice as a doctor you need an active medical professional license from the local governing bodies.

After physicians are licensed, they must renew their license periodically, usually every one or two years, to continue their active status. During this license renewal process, physicians must demonstrate that they have maintained acceptable standards of ethics and medical practice and have not engaged in improper conduct. And in most countries physicians must also show that they have participated in a program of continuing medical education about which I have written in detail in the other chapter of this book.

So if you take a career break from medicine your medical license to practice gets inactivated after one year in most countries. Then once you decide to come back to practice as a doctor again you have to go through all the hassle of doing extensive paperwork and submitting lots of documents again and if your license has been inactive for more than two years, in most countries you may have to sit in an examination which will test that your knowledge it's still up to date to provide safe patient care.

As far as I know, medicine and law are perhaps the only two professions where the professionals are so closely and rigorously monitored and their practice is highly regulated for the right reasons. Public has to have faith and trust in the medical profession and they need to be assured that the doctor they are going to see is a safe doctor. To ensure that, the government and regulating licensing authorities' job is to make the licensing process rigorous and ensure that doctors' knowledge is up to date and Is fit to practice medicine.

So although theoretically its possible for you as a doctor to take a career break and pursue your interest outside the medicine but in reality going through the rigorous process of licensing again to go back into the mainstream medicine and work as doctor again this very thought of going through all the paperwork and possibly sitting in the exam acts as a deterrent to most doctors and their dreams may remain dreams for ever unfortunately.

You may wonder why can't doctors pursue their interest outside medicine when they retire. But you will be surprised to know that most doctors do not want to retire and keep on practicing and caring for their patients as long as they can. I have seen lots of doctors who came back from their retirement to practice again.

But I suppose it depends on the preferences and choices of the individual. After going too far in their professional career lots of doctors may have given up on their dreams or even completely forgotten about it or lost those skills such as playing a musical instrument, and the only way they think they can keep themselves occupied is by practicing medicine which they have been doing through most of their life.

CHAPTER 14

A NEW CHAPTER ABROAD: UNRAVELING THE EXCITEMENT AND CHALLENGES OF RELOCATING FOR A FRESH PROFESSIONAL JOURNEY

A s I have done these three times in my career, and with increasing globalization, I am pretty sure lots of you will do that as well. I really want to touch on this topic, based on my personal experiences.

Relocating to a different country as a doctor is like embarking on an exhilarating adventure with its fair share of pleasure and problems. On the one hand, there's the excitement of immersing yourself in a new culture, exploring unfamiliar landscapes, and embracing diverse medical practices. It's a chance to broaden your horizons and gain a fresh perspective on healthcare.

However, the path is not without its challenges. The process of adapting to a new healthcare system, navigating through bureaucratic hurdles, and obtaining the necessary certifications can be a rollercoaster ride. Language barriers and cultural differences may add a pinch of spice to the mix, making communication a delightful puzzle to solve.

Also to bear in mind that even if you have and active medical license in one country and you have decided to relocate to a different country to practice as a doctor you have to apply and go through the rigorous and lengthy process of obtaining medical license of that particular country which will also include submitting all your qualifications starting from high school to post graduate medical degree.

In most countries this may also require passing and examination conducted by the medical council of that particular country for example in USA it's called United States Medical Licensing Examination (USMLE) and in UK Professional and Linguistic Assessments Board test, known as the PLAB test.

Of course, homesickness and adjusting to a different way of life can be daunting. Finding a sense of belonging in a foreign land may require effort and an open mind. But with resilience, flexibility, and a dash of humor, the journey becomes an opportunity for personal growth and professional development.

Yet, the rewards can be extraordinary. Connecting with patients from different backgrounds, learning from local experts, and witnessing the impact of your skills on a global scale can be immensely fulfilling. You become part of a vibrant international medical community, sharing knowledge and experiences that transcend borders.

Ultimately, relocating as a doctor opens doors to a world of possibilities. It challenges you to embrace the unknown, celebrate diversity, and make a difference in the lives of people far from home.

So, pack your stethoscope and brace yourself for an extraordinary adventure filled with both pleasure and problems. The experiences you gain and the lives you touch will make it all worthwhile. This will be my personal opinion as I have done it several times.

CHAPTER 15

CONQUERING THE IVORY TOWERS - ADMISSION TO THE MEDICAL SCHOOLS - TOUGH BUT DOABLE

"The greatest teacher, failure is." - Star Wars: Episode III - Revenge of the Sith

Admission to medical school no doubt is a highly competitive and rigorous process. It requires dedication, perseverance, and a strong academic foundation. However, while it is undoubtedly challenging, it is also achievable with the right preparation and mindset.

The acceptance rate of medical schools across the world is very low. It could be as low as 3% in Germany and Korea, 10 to 15% in Japan, France and China. It's about 40% in the US, UK and in India. This is as per the data provided by these countries' entrance exam conducting bodies. But of course the percentage varies a lot from one Medical School to another, the most highly rated once having an acceptance rate of only about 10%.

With diligent preparation, a well-rounded application, and a genuine passion for medicine, you can increase your chances of success.

Nowadays, just graduating in medicine is the beginning of many years of training until you sub-specialize in the specialty of your choice. No matter which country you are going to get trained in, it will take on average about ten to twelve years before you can start practicing as an independent sub specialist. Currently there are so many sub specialties to choose from that you may be spoiled with the choices.

When you are planning to choose medicine as your career one of the most important factor for you to keep in mind is that it is a long journey to reach to get to your target or the goal and halfway through you might get frustrated or disillusioned when you will see your other friends who have choose other career pathways such as going into the software engineering and joined top tech companies such as Google, Microsoft or Meta or took economics and then gone into the banking industry.

They will be into the job after graduating within three to four years and by the time you finish graduation and specialization in any field of medicine which is ten years at least they will already be six years into the job and may already be earning high salary and getting promoted to the next level.

Although in medicine after graduating during your postgraduate training you will start getting some stipend but that would be nowhere near to tech companies equivalent salary your friends will be earning. I am trying to compare the students of High School who have the same level of aptitude as students entering into the medical school in which case most of the students going into other professions such as banking and software engineering most likely will be earning more than what post graduate medical students will earn.

CHAPTER 16

CHARTING YOUR COURSE TO MEDICAL MASTERY: HOW CAN YOU PREPARE FOR A CAREER IN MEDICINE

"Remember, every journey starts with a single step. Pursuing a career in medicine is your first step towards a world of endless possibilities."

A s I mentioned earlier in this book, I am not a professional educational counselor, who will be in a better position to guide you regarding your educational requirements at high school and higher secondary level and choosing medicine as a career depending on the country where you are currently studying.

I am going to give here a brief outline of the educational requirements but please do discuss these in detail with the educational counselor of your school.

Before I delve into this topic, it's important to note that the specific requirements and process for becoming a doctor can vary by country and region. It's advisable to research the requirements of the country or region in which you intend to practice medicine for accurate and up-to-date information.

In most countries except the United States of America where you have to do a four year Bachelor's Degree, you can enter into medical school straight after High School diploma or Higher Secondary education. I have to say I used to be quite skeptical about this requirement of doing a graduate degree before entering into medical school. My thought was, why waste four crucial years, while in other countries students will be in their 4th year of medical graduation, the students in the USA will just start their journey on a long and winding road of their medical career.

But now I realize actually completing an undergraduate degree before committing to the career in medicine has distinct advantages.

Pursuing a bachelor's degree allows students to gain a broader education and develop critical thinking skills. Many medical schools value applicants who have a well-rounded education and have explored various academic disciplines beyond the sciences. This broader knowledge base can enhance a student's ability to approach healthcare challenges from different perspectives and adapt to the evolving landscape of medicine.

The undergraduate experience also provides students with opportunities for personal growth, self-discovery, and maturity. It offers a chance to develop essential life skills, such as effective communication, teamwork, leadership, and time management. These skills are invaluable in the medical profession, where doctors need to work collaboratively, communicate effectively with patients and colleagues, and manage complex responsibilities.

And most importantly, completing an undergraduate degree before applying to medical school allows students to explore different fields, gain exposure to diverse disciplines, and make an informed decision about their career choice. Some students may enter college with an interest in medicine but later discover other career paths that better align with their passions and strengths.

If you are reading this book I am resuming that you are already High school or Higher Secondary student with the strong focus on science subjects as your main subjects depending on the country where you are studying currently except United States of America where you will be planning to do a bachelor's degree in science related field such as biology chemistry or biochemistry, commonly known as pre-med amongst the students.

Most countries require students to pass specific entrance examinations or tests as part of the application process for medical school. These exams assess the candidate's knowledge and aptitude for medical studies.

I think it's really useful and helpful for you that while you are studying in High school or Higher Secondary School or for the Bachelor's degree, to shadow a doctor or few doctors of different specialties particularly in the specialty which attracts you for example if you are aspiring to become a brain surgeon, you should shadow and follow a neurosurgeon in your city and observe what is the daily routine of that person on a day to day basis.

Depending on the country where you are currently studying, lots of hospitals, typically government hospitals, have a program called, Observer ship or work experience for the high school students.

However during COVID pandemic because of the health and safety reasons most hospitals withdrew this scheme, which hopefully will be back again soon.

I have been involved with lots of high school students coming for observer ship in the hospitals where I have been working particularly in the United Kingdom. The feedback from the students have been very positive

During observer ship, which is usually between one to four weeks, the students are rotated to different departments in different settings such as outpatient clinics or in patient wards and even Intensive Care units.

I think this is the best way for you to get the correct insight of the medical profession and particularly the life of a doctor.

No matter how many sessions you take with an educational counselor or watch videos on the internet or TV programs related to the medical profession or even reading several books including this one, none of these will be as valuable as shadowing a real doctor.

Some of you may have one or both parents in the medical profession and you may have seen their routine from a very young age as a child but there may be a bias here as your parents may be a positive or negative influence for you. So although it will be a lot easier for you to join Observer ship at a place where your parents are working, there may be a bias so personally I will suggest that you avoid that and follow some other doctor.

I'll give my personal example. My father was a doctor as I have mentioned before, and although I did not intend to become a doctor and wanted to become a movie director but somewhere perhaps subconsciously the medical profession stuck into my brain and I got convinced by closely observing the respect and popularity my father used to get being a doctor that I ended up going into the same profession.

On the contrary, although both myself and my wife are doctors, our both sons decided not to go into medicine. As a child, when they were growing up they only saw lots of time, only one parent being with them at one time to take care of them or even sometimes they had to be with the child minder as both myself and my wife used to work in the shifts during our medical training.

This I feel must have created a negative influence on them and they decided not to choose medicine as a career. I must say that my wife realized this very early on when our kids were very young that she has to choose between the progression of her professional career or the family and kids and she unfortunately has to take long career break to be with our sons to support them mentally and physically for which not only me both of our sons are grateful for her sacrifice.

We know without her sacrifice in the early part of her career we would not have been where we are today.

By telling all that I also wanted to highlight a very important aspect of choosing medicine as a career particularly in reference to the girls who will be mother and wife at some point. They may have to be prepared to take some career break, as the data from UK suggest most of them prefer working part time, which in fact is not a bad thing, as all you are doing is just extending your training perhaps for some more years but the advantage is that you are acting as solid pillar and a foundation for your family, particularly to your kids when they are very young and growing, as this childhood will not come back again and you may regret later on if you have missed them watching growing up. Your career can wait or can be stretched for a few more years and you can still reach the point of your career where you wanted to be with the fulfillment that you managed to balance both your professional and personal life.

Although this was in reference to the girls, there is no reason why boys cannot take a career break to play the role of a responsible and caring husband and father. There are lots of examples of the doctors who have done this to help their wives finish their medical training.

So going back to the observer ship or work experience , if you have managed to do one and you have decided yes this is the career I want to choose then in most countries you have to clear an entrance examination. These entrance exams assess the candidates knowledge and aptitude for medical studies.

> "Choosing medicine is not just about a career; it's about a lifelong commitment to serving others and making a positive difference in the world."

These entrance exams are highly competitive and require you to score at least the cut off for the satisfactory score but higher your score, more are the chances of you getting offers from Medical Schools

Apart from the entrance exams you need to have a very strong academic record during your High school, Higher Secondary School or International Baccalaureate Program.

Process of admission to medical schools also involves in most countries letters of recommendations from your high school teachers and the final step is the interview either by the medical school directly or by the panel of the governing body conducting these examinations

Finally if you successfully pass all the steps, depending on your final score and the results of your High school or IB you will be ranked and based on your ranking Medical Schools will offer you a place.

Whether you are offered a place in the top Medical School of your country or any other Medical School in the list, these colleges must be recognized by the local government and educational authorities.

In my opinion, yes the quality of education may vary from one Medical School to another however you should not be disheartened if you're not offered a place which are top ranked and the one you were aiming for, as this is going to be the foundation stone and stepping stone for embarking on a long journey.

Even if you don't not get the Medical School of your choice, don't worry, just put all your effort to get the knowledge out of that as much as possible and prepare yourself for the next step which is to get the postgraduate training.

The next stop on this journey will be doing a postgraduate or specialized training which Is essential now in no matter which country you are going to practice in as the medicine has become very specialized nowadays and patients are looking mostly for doctors who specialize in a particular specialty even General physicians (GP) in UK or Family Physicians in USA have to go through rigorous specialized training after obtaining MBBS or MBChB Degree which are the graduate degrees.

Postgraduate and specialty training is the most important and penultimate step of a doctor in their career. As I mentioned before in the current era, to get trained in a particular specialty and practice as a specialist is the option you have to take as there is no other option.

Even in the rural areas, if a patient has a problem with their health they want to see a doctor who specializes in the field related to their health issues for example they would prefer to see a pediatrician for their child's fever or a women would like to see a gynecologist for her gynecological issues and not only that she may prefer to see a female doctor although even in smaller towns or even in Middle Eastern countries that barrier is no more and there are very successful and competent male obstetricians and gynecologists.

Name given to the specialty training varies from one country to another, for example in UK and Europe it is called Specialty Training Program, in the US it's known as Residency and Fellowship program and in India, Postgraduate Medical Training, but overall the structure is more less similar.

A mention earlier on that previously many years ago, MBBS doctors will see all category of patients but now, General physicians or Family Physicians do similar kind of job, they see patients of all ages including children and even women's in initial stages of pregnancy and with gynecological problems however the difference now is that these doctor go through a rigorous post graduate training or specialty training where there are rotated through different specialties like surgery, medicine, pediatrics and obstetrics.

They also have to pass an exam before they can get Professional Healthcare License by the licensing authorities.

To get into the post graduate training and specialization in most countries you have to sit again in an entrance or competency based exam which may occur in different stages including the final stage which is an interview and depending on your score and final ranking in the entrance exam you will have a counseling, where you rank would be matched with different specialties and training posts available.

This is the route which medical students have to take to get into specialized training in most countries including the USA, Europe, India and China.

In the UK however there is no entrance exam but you have to go through the interview process to get into the specialty training program except few medical and surgical specialties where you do need to clear an exam to get into a higher training program.

The good thing is that in most countries during your post graduate or specialist training you do get paid, either by the government authorities or by the hospital you are getting trained in.

CHAPTER 17

SURVIVING THE GAUNTLET: GAUNTLET: THE THRILLING TRUTH ABOUT MEDICAL SCHOOL ATTRITION

"It's not how many times you get knocked down that counts, it's how many times you get back up." - Rocky Balboa

E ssentially, the attrition rate measures how many people leave, voluntarily or involuntarily.

Before embarking on the steep and rigorous journey named 'medical school,' it is only natural for you to wonder about the odds of completing and making it to the end of the road. Aside from the graduation rates, it is also necessary for pre-med students to know the medical school dropout rate.

Medical school is akin to a roller coaster, it pulls you through the highest of highs and then drops you to the lowest of lows.

For a rough estimate, the overall dropout rate in medical school is about 10%. However, it is pretty hard to find reliable statistics. The dropout rate for a standard, 4-year program is between 15.7% and 18.4%, as claimed by the Association of American Medical Colleges.

The attrition rate of medical school in the UK is, on average, about 10%. The majority of people who drop out of medical school will do so in the first year.

If you have decided to go into medicine and are fortunate enough to get into medical school then you are amongst the top 10 to 15% of thousands of students in high school or higher secondary who gave entrance examinations. In other words, about 85 to 90% unfortunately could not qualify.

CHAPTER 18

WHY DO MED STUDENTS DROP OUT? UNCOVERING THE KEY FACTORS THAT CONTRIBUTE TO ATTRITION

"Failure is not the opposite of success; it's a stepping stone to success." - Crazy Rich Asians

Surprisingly, as intimidating as med school sounds, most students tend to drop out for non-academic reasons.

Most common reason being making the wrong career choice.

It is not entirely uncommon for med students to realize that they chose the wrong career. It can be challenging for them to accept and stomach that becoming a doctor is not for them, especially if you have the expectation ingrained thoroughly.

Some medical students follow in the footsteps of their doctor parents. While others imagine the prestige of earning the title of doctor, only to discover that they have a chronic case of nerves and squeamishness when dissecting cadavers.

When med students realize that they are not cut out for the profession, they have no other choice but to drop out. That's both money and time wasted.

So, before entering medical school, do some soul-searching to ensure that it is the path you want to take and embark on. Even if you are the most logical person in the world, still spend the time contemplating your reasons for wanting to pursue a career in medicine.

Your very first day in medical school will perhaps be the happiest day of your life and it will indeed be a proud moment for your parents and family. It will also be a moment of pride and sense of achievement for you and all your effort and hard work has translated into success.

But for some of you after a few days or months the reality may kick in and you may start to think that this is not for me but you may not like to share this feeling with your friends or with your parents. You may be more reluctant to talk to your parents particularly if they are doctors themselves and had a dream of their son or daughter becoming a doctor. You would not like to disappoint them or hurt their feelings and this is quite natural.

You may also be thinking that if I drop out from medical school the society will think that I am a loser, who could not handle the hard work and pressure of studies which obviously is quite rigorous in medicine.

For some of you there may be financial pressure as well. Spending years in med school, amassing lots of money in student debt or borrowing money from your parents and devoting the next four or five decades of your life to juggling a fast-paced career, you may realize that this is not for me.

After spending a few months in a medical school, if you really feel that this is not for you and I perhaps made the wrong choice, you may want to get out of it. Just do what your heart says as you do not want to follow a path which will make you sad, frustrated and demoralized for the rest of your life. Leaving Medical School halfway is not the end of your journey neither is the end of the world just think about your happiness.

The fact that you made it to medical school is in fact a testimony itself that you are the brightest brain among your peers and if you choose a different career pathway, there is no reason why you would not succeed. The chances of success will be higher in fact because you will be happier, boosted with lots of good hormones in your body.

For your parents, it may be a shocking news initially that you are deciding to leave medicine but remember, all they want is to see you happy, so in the end they will support your decision wholeheartedly.

CHAPTER 19

RISING FROM THE ASHES: WHAT HAPPENS NEXT AFTER YOU FAIL EXAMS IN MEDICAL SCHOOL ?

"Don't let anyone ever make you feel like you don't deserve what you want." - 10 Things I Hate About You

Failure is not common, because college tutors are usually good at spotting students in difficulty and arranging extra help and there will certainly be additional help from the school if you are in difficulties.

But failures do occur and the pass out rate is rarely 100% in any stage of exams or in different subjects. Some subjects such as anatomy are more dreaded by the students than others.

Medical school curriculum is rigorous and demanding, requiring a significant amount of studying, memorization, and critical thinking. The volume and complexity of the material can be overwhelming for some students, leading to difficulties in keeping up with coursework and exams.

Although the students entering into medical school are bright, hard working students, transitioning from undergraduate studies to the medical school environment can be a significant adjustment. The different teaching methods, high-stakes exams, and increased expectations may require students to develop new study strategies and adapt to the unique learning environment of medical school. Students who adapt to these quickly have no problems in passing their exams.

Medical schools are different from other professional colleges. Here apart from the academic workload you will also have other responsibilities, such as clinical rotations, research, and extracurricular activities, and balancing out all these can be challenging. Poor time management skills or difficulty prioritizing tasks may result in inadequate preparation for exams or difficulty meeting deadlines.

Students are generally permitted to fail at least one exam while studying at medical school. The exact policy regarding a student who's failed will vary from medical school to medical school but broadly they will be allowed to re-sit the exam for a second time before further measures are taken.

And this is true in all the medical schools in most countries.

Because a normal undergraduate science degree takes three years, and medical school is generally five years long, if a medical student has completed at least three years of the course before dropping out they normally get to leave with a BSc or equivalent in some countries like the UK but this option is not available in most other countries.

CHAPTER 20

PRESCRIBING PRECISION: MASTERING THE ART OF MINIMIZING HUMAN ERRORS IN MEDICINE

"To err is human, but errors can be prevented."

Nowadays Healthcare is compared with the Aviation industry which works on zero error policy. And rightly so, Health Care should also try to reduce the incidence of clinical errors as much as possible to bring down the incidence of mobility and mortality due to human errors.

It is really important to understand that we are talking about human errors here. In the aviation industry pilots spend hours in a virtual cockpit before they can fly a real aircraft and that too as a co-pilot with senior pilots.

If we try to compare that with healthcare, although doctors are also doing simulation training where they are given different scenarios and dummy patient or a mannequin, which thanks to the brilliant advances in technology, behave like a real patient and all the parameters such as blood pressure, heartbeat and breathing, which are all controlled by a remote by the team who is conducting these training.

Personally I feel this is the best way to improve the quality of teamwork, reduce the chances of human error and consequently reduce the morbidity and mortality of our patients. When faced with a real patient, the doctors and nurses reaction and response in similar scenarios will be much quicker with less degree of anxiety, as they have faced the same scenario several times during their stimulation drills and this is particularly very important during emergency situations, resuscitating a patient.

I was recently approached by a tech company, which is using virtual reality (VR) headsets such as Oculus, which you guys must be knowing very well as it is quite popular in the virtual gaming industry. This startup company, which is based in the UK, is growing very fast and is selling its products to various hospitals in Europe and USA.

VR simulation has been integral to training in aviation and industrial safety for nearly thirty years. Thankfully It has now become a proven force in healthcare increasing safety, visibility, and reproducibility of actions as well as reducing costs of training.

Apart from emergency medicine where of course it is very useful, one other specialty where its finding its use is for surgical trainees. Virtual reality simulated training can teach vital skills to surgeons before they take patients under the knife.

I want to see this simulation training for healthcare professionals like pilots to become a mandatory part of professional licensing requirements.

The benefits of VR simulation in healthcare are also evidence based, there are lots of studies proving its benefits in training doctors at various levels.

CHAPTER 21

THE SILENT STRUGGLE: UNMASKING THE UNTOLD STORIES OF MENTAL HEALTH IN THE HEALING PROFESSION

"It's not what happens to you, but how you react to it that matters." - The Pursuit of Happyness

Mental health of the doctors during and post COVID-19 particularly has taken a hit.

If we look at the data from Survey Healthcare Global (SHG), which was sourced in February 14-16, 2022 from six of the most pandemic-impacted medical specialties in the US, UK, France, Germany, Italy and Spain.

This report on the mental health of healthcare professionals (HCPs) in six Western nations shows that chronic staffing shortages are impacting both patient care and patient mental health, as well as physician mental health.

A third (34%) of responding physicians say they have observed an increase in medical errors as a result of staff shortages, at a high of 58% in Spain.

34% of Doctors Worldwide Observed Increased Medical Errors Due to Staffing Shortages, as their mental health suffers, says Survey Healthcare Global Report.

75% of HCPs in US, UK, and EU nations feel stressed. In Spainthey faced the highest levels of stress and anxiety, over 50% considered leaving medicine in past three months.

"You don't have to be perfect to be amazing." -
Frozen

There are various reasons for this rise amongst doctors.

Stress and Burnout being the most common, this was the main factor particularly during COVID-19 pandemic. Doctors face high levels of stress due to long working hours, heavy workloads, and the emotional toll of dealing with patients' suffering. These pressures can obviously contribute to burnout, which is characterized by emotional exhaustion, depersonalization, and a reduced sense of accomplishment. Burnout then as consequence can significantly impact mental well-being.

Doctors often face emotionally challenging situations, such as delivering difficult diagnoses, witnessing patient suffering, or dealing with patient deaths. The emotional demands of the profession can accumulate and lead to compassion fatigue, vicarious trauma, and increased vulnerability to mental health issues.

The demanding nature of medical careers can create challenges in maintaining a healthy work-life balance. Long hours, irregular schedules, and the need for continuous professional development can leave little time for self-care, relaxation, and meaningful personal relationships, which are essential for mental well-being.

And last but not the least, despite the growing awareness of mental health, there is still a significant stigma surrounding mental health issues, particularly in the medical fraternity. Many doctors fear negative repercussions on their professional reputation or career advancement if they disclose their mental health struggles, leading to reluctance in seeking help or support.

But on the positive side, all these factors can be effectively dealt with. Doctors, regulating authorities and hospital management are all trying to address these issues as it's in everybody's interest that we don't lose such scarce and highly qualified professionals. After all, it takes years to train a doctor, who cannot be replaced in one day.

CHAPTER 22

NAVIGATING THE HIGH-STAKES WORLD OF LITIGATIONS AGAINST DOCTORS

Being a doctor is like performing a high-wire act without a safety net, while juggling angry cats. One wrong move, and you might end up in a courtroom, trying to convince a jury that you didn't mix up your stethoscope with a kazoo. But, at least it keeps the lawyers entertained!

Every doctor within the limits of their expertise wants to help their patients and wants the best outcome and has every intention to do so.

If you are going to choose medicine as a career, this is one thing you should be aware of. In spite of all the good intentions to treat his or her patient, there has been a significant increase in litigation against the doctors.

I will give you some data to back up this statement.

A study published in the New England Journal of Medicine in 2011 analyzed malpractice claims in the United States over a five-year period and found that approximately 7.6% of physicians faced a malpractice claim each year.

The NHS Litigation Authority in the UK (now known as NHS Resolution) handles claims and litigation against healthcare providers in the NHS, UK.. According to their annual reports, the number of clinical negligence claims received has been steadily increasing over the years. For example, in the 2019/2020 financial year, NHS Resolution received 10,678 new clinical negligence claims.

The MPS is a medical defense organization that provides professional indemnity to healthcare professionals in the UK. They publish reports and data on medical litigation trends. According to their report "The Changing Face of Medical Malpractice Claims," the number of medical malpractice claims in the UK has been increasing over the past decade.

I have to say that even when lawsuits are not

successful or are resolved in favor of the physician, the litigation process can still have significant emotional and financial impacts on doctors. The stress of litigation and potential reputational damage are factors that can affect healthcare professionals involved in malpractice claims.

CHAPTER 23

THE COURTROOM CHRONICLES: UNVEILING THE SURGE IN LITIGATIONS AGAINST DOCTORS

There are various reasons as to why they are increasing. Important ones are the higher expectations of the public and patients for the standard of care they receive. Any perceived deviation from these expectations leads to higher likelihood of litigation.

With the passage of every decade the society and the lifestyle changes. When I started practicing medicine nearly thirty-five years ago and during the initial years of my medical training, both in India and in the UK there were no mobile phones, the internet just came but was not easily available to the public and was very expensive.

So I would say during the pre internet and mobile phone era the patients will completely trust the doctors and health care professionals and will follow their advice religiously because they had no reasons to question their expertise and wisdom. The trust factor was very high.

But that did not mean that doctors were taking patients for granted and were not sharing all the information with their patients or hiding anything from them which they can now find on the Internet. Doctors have always been honest to their patients, they try to give good quality services. Vast majority of doctors in any era have always been treating their patients with good intentions and put all their efforts into making their patients better and healthier.

In pre pre-internet and mobile phone era the people's lifestyle was more relaxed. As they were socializing more and communicating more directly with human beings, they were able to share their anxieties and concerns first with their friends and families and then with their own doctors. As they would trust their doctors more in those times, they were feeling more reassured and that was definitely bringing down their anxiety levels.

I suppose it's very hard for me to convince you guys of this generation for whom it will be hard to imagine the world and life without mobile phones and access to the internet.

CHAPTER 24

THE DANCE OF SAFETY: EXPLORING THE SYMBIOTIC RELATIONSHIP BETWEEN DOCTORS AND PATIENTS

"Caring for those who care for us is a duty we all share. Ensuring the safety and well-being of doctors is not just a necessity, but

a moral imperative."

The patients are not always obliging and grateful - this is the statement given by one of the medical students.

As more than 50% of the world's population lives in Africa, India and China, students currently studying in these countries and aspiring to become doctors must also consider the safety concerns when they start practicing as a doctor.

When you manage a critically ill patient the emotions of the closed family members are very high and if the patient doesn't respond to treatment and sadly dies, although in most of the cases it's not doctors or nurses fault but the close family members take out all their anger and frustration on the health care team and they may even be physically abusive to them.

But there are ways by which doctors can handle these situations better and prioritize their safety.

Clear and effective communication is most important and crucial in maintaining a safe work environment. As in my experience, poor communication between doctors and patients is number one factor leading unfortunately towards verbal and even rarely to physical abuse towards the doctors.

Doctors should not only communicate well with their patients but also openly with their colleagues, supervisors, and staff, sharing concerns, reporting incidents, and discussing potential safety issues to promote a culture of safety and collaboration.

Every hospital has and should have very strict policies against any kind of abuse towards healthcare professionals, which is completely unacceptable.

Doctors should also be aware of their surroundings and take necessary precautions to maintain personal security. This may include being mindful of personal belongings, using secure parking areas, and following institutional security protocols.

CHAPTER 25

TO RETIRE OR NOT TO RETIRE: THE DOCTOR'S DILEMMA - DECIDING WHEN TO HANG UP THE STETHOSCOPE

While many doctors choose to continue practicing, retirement decisions are highly individual and depend on a variety of personal, professional, and financial factors. Some doctors may choose to retire earlier or transition into different roles, while others may continue practicing well into their later years. Ultimately, the decision to retire or continue working is a personal one based on individual circumstances and preferences.

Although as I mentioned there are several reasons why some doctors may not choose to retire at all, the two important ones I think are, being a doctor forms a significant part of a person's identity. The role and status that come with being a doctor can be deeply ingrained, making it difficult to let go of that identity and transition into retirement.

Doctors often develop long-term relationships with patients, colleagues, and staff members over the course of their careers. These relationships can be fulfilling and provide a sense of community and connection, which may contribute to the decision to continue practicing.

I see now the trend is changing and lots of doctors, who do not want to give up the medical profession completely are opting for part-time practice to allow them to maintain a better work-life balance. This allows them to continue practicing medicine while also having more time for personal pursuits, hobbies, or spending time with family and loved ones.

Mentorship and teaching by very experienced doctors who would be keen to pass on their knowledge and skills to the next generation of healthcare professionals, will be my favorite option. They may take on roles as mentors, educators, or consultants, contributing to the development and growth of future healthcare providers. This invaluable passage of knowledge to younger doctors is something which they may not be able to get by reading textbooks or from internet sources.

CHAPTER 26

FOLLOW YOUR HEARTBEAT: PURSUING MEDICINE WHILE PRIORITIZING YOUR HAPPINESS

"Your work is going to fill a large part of your life, and the only way to be truly satisfied is to do what you believe is great work. And the only way to do great work is to love what you do." - Steve Jobs

In the end, my advice for all of you would be to pursue your passion for medicine while emphasizing the importance of prioritizing your own happiness. A fulfilling career in medicine is only possible when aligned with personal well-being and fulfillment.

So listen to your hearts, explore your interests, and make choices that will lead to a career that brings both professional satisfaction and personal happiness.

ABOUT THE AUTHOR

Dr Mudit Kumar

Dr Mudit Kumar was born in India. He obtained his medical undergraduate MBBS degree and later on did his postgraduate training and specialization in pediatrics and neonatology from the Institute of Medical Sciences, Banaras Hindu University (BHU), India, which has been rated India's 5th best for medical education in the National Institutional Ranking Framework (NIRF) rankings-2022 released by the Ministry of Education, India

He then moved to United Kingdom where he did further training in Pediatrics and Neonatology and worked as Consultant in Pediatrics in National Health Services (NHS) UK

Apart from holding an MD degree, Dr Kumar is also Fellow of Royal College of Pediatrics and child health (FRCPCH) of UK.

Dr Kumar is very keen in teaching medical students

and pediatric trainees. He is also senior examiner for MRCPCH UK exams and part of the group of senior examiners which prepare and write questions for theory and clinical examination conducted by RCPCH UK. He has also been the examiner for Oxford medical school, UK undergraduate exams.

Outside medicine Dr Kumar Is a Movie buff.

Dr Kumar's spouse, Dr Vinita is also a doctor who works with children with Autism. He has two sons, both are graduates. The elder, Shubhrant is pursuing a career in law in the USA and the younger one, Sudhansh is a Mathematician and a gifted musician currently living in London UK.

Printed in Great Britain
by Amazon

24888645R10106